MW01170942

City – State – Country:

Phone Number and Email:

Physician and Contact Information:

Emergency Contact Person and Phone Number:

WHAT IS CONTACT TRACING?

Contact tracing is a public health strategy used to interrupt the spreading of an infectious disease. It begins with talking to the "person of interest" and finding out who they had close contact with in the past several weeks. It then traces those contacts, has them tested for the infection, and treats them. This process is then repeated with each contact exposed to the infection. Contact tracing supports the public health goal of reducing infections in a community.

The goals of contact tracing are:

- To interrupt the transmission patterns thus reducing the spread of an infection in the community;
- To alert "persons of interest" to the possibility of infection and then offer proactive and preventive counseling;
- To offer diagnosis, counseling, and treatment to infected individuals;
- To prevent the person from being infected again if possible;
- To learn more about how a disease impacts a specific community and this knowledge helps to manage and contain how a disease spreads.

Contact tracing is a critical step for disease control in public health. It manages the spread of a disease by addressing community transmission. Historically, disease epidemics and pandemics – such as Smallpox, Tuberculosis, Ebola, HIV, Measles, and SARS – were greatly managed by using exhaustive contact tracing efforts that located all infected individuals and their contacts.

For contact tracing to be effective, the majority of a community needs to participate in the effort.

ABOUT THE AUTHORS & LOG

This logbook was written by Dr. J.A. Talkington who earned a PhD in Environmental Science. Dr. Talkington has also studied disease symptomatology, toxicology, graphic design, and historical research methods. Dr. Talkington is known as a science historian, a business professor, a health researcher, and a certified contact tracer.

The co-author, Dr. N. S. Najd, earned a PhD in Industrial Engineering and Management. Dr. Najd has also studied civil and environmental engineering, systems thinking, English, Arabic, and French. Dr. Najd is known as a project manager, an interdisciplinary professor, and a certified contact tracer.

This logbook was conceived by Dr. Talkington after an email exchange discussing contact tracing with a researcher at the Centers for Disease Control (CDC). It is vital for the 'person of interest' to be able to identify who they have been in contact with during the previous several weeks.

If the 'person of interest' cannot recall all of their interactions, critical information will be lost and the public will be endangered further. Given the privacy concerns about using cellular telephone data to monitor users' movements, a paperback logbook seemed a logical and necessary solution. Recognizing the need, Dr. Talkington created the *Contact Tracing Log – A Logical Necessity*™.

This book allows a person to log vital information about their travels and their interactions with other people. The *Contact Tracing Log – A Logical Necessity*™ is available as a paperback book in multiple sizes on Amazon websites worldwide.

SAMPLE

PLACE and address   **DATE:**   7/4/2020

Eskimo Joe's Restaurant™
DUCK AND ELM - STILLWATER, OKLAHOMA

your health:
Dandy!

NAMES include people you traveled with   **mask on others**

Mike L. - lunch guest.   Y

Bill S. - lunch guest.   N

Alicia - waitress.   Y

other diners   > 6 ft   Y

     about half

describe the social distancing

ARRIVAL TIME   🕐   10:55   (AM) PM

DEPARTURE TIME   🕐   12:30   AM (PM)

transportation 🚶🚴🚗✈️	Drove Ford F250
washed hands before	(yes) - no
hand sanitizer before	yes - (no)
mask on you	(yes) - no
body temperature	98.6
air circulation	outdoors or (inside)
number of people	10-15
washed hands after	yes - (no)
hand sanitizer after	(yes) - no

PLACE and address   DATE:

your health:

NAMES include people you traveled with   **mask yes / no**

—

—

—

—

describe the social distancing

ARRIVAL TIME   AM / PM

DEPARTURE TIME   AM / PM

transportation

washed hands before   yes - no

hand sanitizer before   yes - no

mask on you   yes - no

body temperature

air circulation   outdoors or inside

number of people

washed hands after   yes - no

hand sanitizer after   yes - no

PLACE and address
DATE:

your health:

NAMES include people you traveled with
mask yes / no

___

___

___

___

describe the social distancing

ARRIVAL TIME
AM / PM

DEPARTURE TIME
AM / PM

transportation

washed hands before
yes - no

hand sanitizer before
yes - no

mask on you
yes - no

body temperature

air circulation
outdoors or inside

number of people

washed hands after
yes - no

hand sanitizer after
yes - no

PLACE and address

DATE:

your health:

NAMES include people you traveled with

mask yes / no

___

___

___

___

describe the social distancing

ARRIVAL TIME AM / PM

DEPARTURE TIME AM / PM

transportation

washed hands before — yes - no

hand sanitizer before — yes - no

mask on you — yes - no

body temperature

air circulation — outdoors or inside

number of people

washed hands after — yes - no

hand sanitizer after — yes - no

PLACE and address   DATE:

your health:

NAMES include people you traveled with   **mask yes / no**

___

___

___

___

describe the social distancing

ARRIVAL TIME   AM / PM

DEPARTURE TIME   AM / PM

transportation

washed hands before   yes - no

hand sanitizer before   yes - no

mask on you   yes - no

body temperature

air circulation   outdoors or inside

number of people

washed hands after   yes - no

hand sanitizer after   yes - no

PLACE and address

DATE:

your health:

NAMES include people you traveled with

mask yes / no

___

___

___

___

describe the social distancing

ARRIVAL TIME   AM / PM

DEPARTURE TIME   AM / PM

transportation

washed hands before yes - no

hand sanitizer before yes - no

mask on you yes - no

body temperature

air circulation outdoors or inside

number of people

washed hands after yes - no

hand sanitizer after yes - no

PLACE and address

DATE:

your health:

NAMES include people you traveled with

mask yes / no

___

___

___

___

describe the social distancing

ARRIVAL TIME AM / PM

DEPARTURE TIME AM / PM

transportation

washed hands before — yes - no

hand sanitizer before — yes - no

mask on you — yes - no

body temperature

air circulation — outdoors or inside

number of people

washed hands after — yes - no

hand sanitizer after — yes - no

PLACE and address
DATE:

your health:

NAMES include people you traveled with

mask yes / no

___

___

___

___

describe the social distancing

ARRIVAL TIME   AM / PM

DEPARTURE TIME   AM / PM

transportation

washed hands before yes - no

hand sanitizer before yes - no

mask on you yes - no

body temperature

air circulation outdoors or inside

number of people

washed hands after yes - no

hand sanitizer after yes - no

PLACE and address   **DATE:**

your health:

NAMES include people you traveled with   **mask yes / no**

___

___

___

___

describe the social distancing

ARRIVAL TIME 🕐   AM / PM

DEPARTURE TIME 🕐   AM / PM

transportation 🚶 🚴 🚗

washed hands before   yes - no

hand sanitizer before   yes - no

mask on you   yes - no

body temperature

air circulation   outdoors or inside

number of people

washed hands after   yes - no

hand sanitizer after   yes - no

PLACE and address   **DATE:**

your health:

NAMES include people you traveled with   **mask yes / no**

___

___

___

___

describe the social distancing

ARRIVAL TIME   AM / PM

DEPARTURE TIME   AM / PM

transportation

washed hands before   yes - no

hand sanitizer before   yes - no

mask on you   yes - no

body temperature

air circulation   outdoors or inside

number of people

washed hands after   yes - no

hand sanitizer after   yes - no

PLACE and address

DATE:

your health:

NAMES include people you traveled with

mask yes / no

___

___

___

___

describe the social distancing

ARRIVAL TIME 🕐   AM / PM

DEPARTURE TIME 🕐   AM / PM

transportation

washed hands before   yes - no

hand sanitizer before   yes - no

mask on you   yes - no

body temperature

air circulation   outdoors or inside

number of people

washed hands after   yes - no

hand sanitizer after   yes - no

PLACE and address   DATE:

your health:

NAMES include people you traveled with   **mask yes / no**

___

___

___

___

describe the social distancing

ARRIVAL TIME   AM / PM

DEPARTURE TIME   AM / PM

transportation

washed hands before   yes - no

hand sanitizer before   yes - no

mask on you   yes - no

body temperature

air circulation   outdoors or inside

number of people

washed hands after   yes - no

hand sanitizer after   yes - no

PLACE and address   DATE:

your health:

NAMES include people you traveled with   **mask yes / no**

___

___

___

___

describe the social distancing

ARRIVAL TIME   AM / PM

DEPARTURE TIME   AM / PM

transportation

washed hands before   yes - no

hand sanitizer before   yes - no

mask on you   yes - no

body temperature

air circulation   outdoors or inside

number of people

washed hands after   yes - no

hand sanitizer after   yes - no

PLACE and address

DATE:

your health:

NAMES include people you traveled with

mask yes / no

———

———

———

———

describe the social distancing

ARRIVAL TIME AM / PM

DEPARTURE TIME AM / PM

transportation

washed hands before — yes - no

hand sanitizer before — yes - no

mask on you — yes - no

body temperature

air circulation — outdoors or inside

number of people

washed hands after — yes - no

hand sanitizer after — yes - no

PLACE and address   DATE:

your health:

NAMES include people you traveled with   **mask yes / no**

___

___

___

___

describe the social distancing

ARRIVAL TIME   AM / PM

DEPARTURE TIME   AM / PM

transportation

washed hands before   yes - no

hand sanitizer before   yes - no

mask on you   yes - no

body temperature

air circulation   outdoors or inside

number of people

washed hands after   yes - no

hand sanitizer after   yes - no

PLACE and address
DATE:

your health:

NAMES include people you traveled with
mask yes / no

___

___

___

___

describe the social distancing

ARRIVAL TIME   AM / PM

DEPARTURE TIME   AM / PM

transportation

washed hands before   yes - no

hand sanitizer before   yes - no

mask on you   yes - no

body temperature

air circulation   outdoors or inside

number of people

washed hands after   yes - no

hand sanitizer after   yes - no

PLACE and address   DATE:

your health:

NAMES include people you traveled with   **mask yes / no**

___

___

___

___

describe the social distancing

ARRIVAL TIME 🕐		AM / PM
DEPARTURE TIME 🕐		AM / PM
transportation		
washed hands before		yes - no
hand sanitizer before		yes - no
mask on you		yes - no
body temperature		
air circulation		outdoors or inside
number of people		
washed hands after		yes - no
hand sanitizer after		yes - no

PLACE and address   **DATE:**

your health:

NAMES include people you traveled with   **mask yes / no**

___

___

___

___

describe the social distancing

ARRIVAL TIME	AM / PM
DEPARTURE TIME	AM / PM
transportation	
washed hands before	yes - no
hand sanitizer before	yes - no
mask on you	yes - no
body temperature	
air circulation	outdoors or inside
number of people	
washed hands after	yes - no
hand sanitizer after	yes - no

PLACE and address

DATE:

your health:

NAMES include people you traveled with

mask yes / no

___

___

___

___

describe the social distancing

ARRIVAL TIME 🕐   AM / PM

DEPARTURE TIME 🕐   AM / PM

transportation 🚶 🚴 🚗

washed hands before   yes - no

hand sanitizer before   yes - no

mask on you   yes - no

body temperature

air circulation   outdoors or inside

number of people

washed hands after   yes - no

hand sanitizer after   yes - no

PLACE and address   DATE:

your health:

NAMES include people you traveled with   mask yes / no

___

___

___

___

describe the social distancing

ARRIVAL TIME   AM / PM

DEPARTURE TIME   AM / PM

transportation

washed hands before   yes - no

hand sanitizer before   yes - no

mask on you   yes - no

body temperature

air circulation   outdoors or inside

number of people

washed hands after   yes - no

hand sanitizer after   yes - no

PLACE and address

DATE:

your health:

NAMES include people you traveled with

mask yes / no

___

___

___

___

describe the social distancing

ARRIVAL TIME   AM / PM

DEPARTURE TIME   AM / PM

transportation

washed hands before   yes - no

hand sanitizer before   yes - no

mask on you   yes - no

body temperature

air circulation   outdoors or inside

number of people

washed hands after   yes - no

hand sanitizer after   yes - no

PLACE and address   DATE:

your health:

NAMES include people you traveled with   mask yes / no

___

___

___

___

describe the social distancing

ARRIVAL TIME	AM / PM
DEPARTURE TIME	AM / PM
transportation	
washed hands before	yes - no
hand sanitizer before	yes - no
mask on you	yes - no
body temperature	
air circulation	outdoors or inside
number of people	
washed hands after	yes - no
hand sanitizer after	yes - no

PLACE and address   DATE:

your health:

NAMES include people you traveled with   **mask yes / no**

___

___

___

___

describe the social distancing

ARRIVAL TIME   AM / PM

DEPARTURE TIME   AM / PM

transportation

washed hands before   yes - no

hand sanitizer before   yes - no

mask on you   yes - no

body temperature

air circulation   outdoors or inside

number of people

washed hands after   yes - no

hand sanitizer after   yes - no

PLACE and address   DATE:

your health:

NAMES include people you traveled with   **mask yes / no**

___

___

___

___

describe the social distancing

ARRIVAL TIME   AM / PM

DEPARTURE TIME   AM / PM

transportation

washed hands before   yes - no

hand sanitizer before   yes - no

mask on you   yes - no

body temperature

air circulation   outdoors or inside

number of people

washed hands after   yes - no

hand sanitizer after   yes - no

PLACE and address

DATE:

your health:

NAMES include people you traveled with

mask yes / no

___

___

___

___

describe the social distancing

ARRIVAL TIME	AM / PM
DEPARTURE TIME	AM / PM
transportation	
washed hands before	yes - no
hand sanitizer before	yes - no
mask on you	yes - no
body temperature	
air circulation	outdoors or inside
number of people	
washed hands after	yes - no
hand sanitizer after	yes - no

PLACE and address   DATE:

your health:

NAMES include people you traveled with   **mask yes / no**

___

___

___

___

describe the social distancing

ARRIVAL TIME   AM / PM

DEPARTURE TIME   AM / PM

transportation

washed hands before   yes - no

hand sanitizer before   yes - no

mask on you   yes - no

body temperature

air circulation   outdoors or inside

number of people

washed hands after   yes - no

hand sanitizer after   yes - no

PLACE and address   DATE:

your health:

NAMES include people you traveled with   mask yes / no

___

___

___

___

describe the social distancing

ARRIVAL TIME 🕐   AM / PM

DEPARTURE TIME 🕐   AM / PM

transportation 🚶 🚴 🚗

washed hands before   yes - no

hand sanitizer before   yes - no

mask on you   yes - no

body temperature

air circulation   outdoors or inside

number of people

washed hands after   yes - no

hand sanitizer after   yes - no

PLACE and address　　　**DATE:**

your health:

NAMES include people you traveled with　　　**mask yes / no**

———

———

———

———

describe the social distancing

ARRIVAL TIME 　　　AM / PM

DEPARTURE TIME 　　　AM / PM

transportation

washed hands before　　　yes - no

hand sanitizer before　　　yes - no

mask on you　　　yes - no

body temperature

air circulation　　　outdoors or inside

number of people

washed hands after　　　yes - no

hand sanitizer after　　　yes - no

PLACE and address   DATE:

your health:

NAMES include people you traveled with   mask yes / no

___

___

___

___

describe the social distancing

ARRIVAL TIME 🕐   AM / PM

DEPARTURE TIME 🕐   AM / PM

transportation

washed hands before   yes - no

hand sanitizer before   yes - no

mask on you   yes - no

body temperature

air circulation   outdoors or inside

number of people

washed hands after   yes - no

hand sanitizer after   yes - no

PLACE and address   DATE:

your health:

NAMES include people you traveled with   **mask yes / no**

___

___

___

___

describe the social distancing

ARRIVAL TIME   AM / PM

DEPARTURE TIME   AM / PM

transportation

washed hands before   yes - no

hand sanitizer before   yes - no

mask on you   yes - no

body temperature

air circulation   outdoors or inside

number of people

washed hands after   yes - no

hand sanitizer after   yes - no

PLACE and address

DATE:

your health:

NAMES include people you traveled with

mask yes / no

___

___

___

___

describe the social distancing

ARRIVAL TIME 🕐 AM / PM

DEPARTURE TIME 🕐 AM / PM

transportation

washed hands before | yes - no

hand sanitizer before | yes - no

mask on you | yes - no

body temperature

air circulation | outdoors or inside

number of people

washed hands after | yes - no

hand sanitizer after | yes - no

PLACE and address

DATE:

your health:

NAMES include people you traveled with

mask yes / no

___

___

___

___

describe the social distancing

ARRIVAL TIME 　　　　AM / PM

DEPARTURE TIME 　　　　AM / PM

transportation

washed hands before　　　　yes - no

hand sanitizer before　　　　yes - no

mask on you　　　　yes - no

body temperature

air circulation　　　　outdoors or inside

number of people

washed hands after　　　　yes - no

hand sanitizer after　　　　yes - no

PLACE and address

DATE:

your health:

NAMES include people you traveled with

mask yes / no

___

___

___

___

describe the social distancing

ARRIVAL TIME 🕐   AM / PM

DEPARTURE TIME 🕐   AM / PM

transportation

washed hands before   yes - no

hand sanitizer before   yes - no

mask on you   yes - no

body temperature

air circulation   outdoors or inside

number of people

washed hands after   yes - no

hand sanitizer after   yes - no

PLACE and address   **DATE:**

your health:

NAMES include people you traveled with   **mask yes / no**

___

___

___

___

describe the social distancing

ARRIVAL TIME   AM / PM

DEPARTURE TIME   AM / PM

transportation

washed hands before   yes - no

hand sanitizer before   yes - no

mask on you   yes - no

body temperature

air circulation   outdoors or inside

number of people

washed hands after   yes - no

hand sanitizer after   yes - no

PLACE and address

DATE:

your health:

NAMES include people you traveled with

mask yes / no

___

___

___

___

describe the social distancing

ARRIVAL TIME	AM / PM
DEPARTURE TIME	AM / PM
transportation	
washed hands before	yes - no
hand sanitizer before	yes - no
mask on you	yes - no
body temperature	
air circulation	outdoors or inside
number of people	
washed hands after	yes - no
hand sanitizer after	yes - no

PLACE and address

DATE:

your health:

NAMES include people you traveled with

mask yes / no

____

____

____

____

describe the social distancing

ARRIVAL TIME   AM / PM

DEPARTURE TIME   AM / PM

transportation

washed hands before   yes - no

hand sanitizer before   yes - no

mask on you   yes - no

body temperature

air circulation   outdoors or inside

number of people

washed hands after   yes - no

hand sanitizer after   yes - no

PLACE and address

DATE:

your health:

NAMES include people you traveled with

mask yes / no

___

___

___

___

describe the social distancing

ARRIVAL TIME   AM / PM

DEPARTURE TIME   AM / PM

transportation

washed hands before   yes - no

hand sanitizer before   yes - no

mask on you   yes - no

body temperature

air circulation   outdoors or inside

number of people

washed hands after   yes - no

hand sanitizer after   yes - no

PLACE and address   DATE:

your health:

NAMES include people you traveled with   **mask yes / no**

——

——

——

——

describe the social distancing

ARRIVAL TIME   AM / PM

DEPARTURE TIME   AM / PM

transportation

washed hands before   yes - no

hand sanitizer before   yes - no

mask on you   yes - no

body temperature

air circulation   outdoors or inside

number of people

washed hands after   yes - no

hand sanitizer after   yes - no

Contact Tracing LOG: A Logical Necessity™ Copyright © 2020 J.A. Talkington & N.S. Najd

PLACE and address

DATE:

your health:

NAMES include people you traveled with

mask yes / no

___

___

___

___

describe the social distancing

ARRIVAL TIME   AM / PM

DEPARTURE TIME   AM / PM

transportation

washed hands before   yes - no

hand sanitizer before   yes - no

mask on you   yes - no

body temperature

air circulation   outdoors or inside

number of people

washed hands after   yes - no

hand sanitizer after   yes - no

PLACE and address   DATE:

your health:

NAMES include people you traveled with   **mask yes / no**

—

—

—

—

describe the social distancing

ARRIVAL TIME   AM / PM

DEPARTURE TIME   AM / PM

transportation

washed hands before   yes - no

hand sanitizer before   yes - no

mask on you   yes - no

body temperature

air circulation   outdoors or inside

number of people

washed hands after   yes - no

hand sanitizer after   yes - no

PLACE and address   DATE:

your health:

NAMES include people you traveled with   **mask yes / no**

___

___

___

___

describe the social distancing

ARRIVAL TIME   AM / PM

DEPARTURE TIME   AM / PM

transportation

washed hands before   yes - no

hand sanitizer before   yes - no

mask on you   yes - no

body temperature

air circulation   outdoors or inside

number of people

washed hands after   yes - no

hand sanitizer after   yes - no

PLACE and address   DATE:

your health:

NAMES include people you traveled with   **mask yes / no**

———

———

———

———

describe the social distancing

ARRIVAL TIME   AM / PM

DEPARTURE TIME   AM / PM

transportation

washed hands before   yes - no

hand sanitizer before   yes - no

mask on you   yes - no

body temperature

air circulation   outdoors or inside

number of people

washed hands after   yes - no

hand sanitizer after   yes - no

PLACE and address

DATE:

your health:

NAMES include people you traveled with

mask yes / no

___

___

___

___

describe the social distancing

ARRIVAL TIME AM / PM

DEPARTURE TIME AM / PM

transportation

washed hands before | yes - no

hand sanitizer before | yes - no

mask on you | yes - no

body temperature

air circulation | outdoors or inside

number of people

washed hands after | yes - no

hand sanitizer after | yes - no

PLACE and address   DATE:

your health:

NAMES include people you traveled with   **mask yes / no**

___

___

___

___

describe the social distancing

ARRIVAL TIME   AM / PM

DEPARTURE TIME   AM / PM

transportation

washed hands before   yes - no

hand sanitizer before   yes - no

mask on you   yes - no

body temperature

air circulation   outdoors or inside

number of people

washed hands after   yes - no

hand sanitizer after   yes - no

PLACE and address   DATE:

your health:

NAMES include people you traveled with   **mask yes / no**

___

___

___

___

describe the social distancing

ARRIVAL TIME   AM / PM

DEPARTURE TIME   AM / PM

transportation

washed hands before   yes - no

hand sanitizer before   yes - no

mask on you   yes - no

body temperature

air circulation   outdoors or inside

number of people

washed hands after   yes - no

hand sanitizer after   yes - no

PLACE and address   **DATE:**

your health:

NAMES include people you traveled with   **mask yes / no**

___

___

___

___

describe the social distancing

ARRIVAL TIME   AM / PM

DEPARTURE TIME   AM / PM

transportation

washed hands before   yes - no

hand sanitizer before   yes - no

mask on you   yes - no

body temperature

air circulation   outdoors or inside

number of people

washed hands after   yes - no

hand sanitizer after   yes - no

PLACE and address

DATE:

your health:

NAMES include people you traveled with

mask yes / no

___

___

___

___

describe the social distancing

ARRIVAL TIME 　　　AM / PM

DEPARTURE TIME 　　　AM / PM

transportation

washed hands before　　　yes - no

hand sanitizer before　　　yes - no

mask on you　　　yes - no

body temperature

air circulation　　　outdoors or inside

number of people

washed hands after　　　yes - no

hand sanitizer after　　　yes - no

PLACE and address

DATE:

your health:

NAMES include people you traveled with

mask yes / no

___

___

___

___

describe the social distancing

ARRIVAL TIME 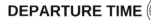 AM / PM

DEPARTURE TIME AM / PM

transportation

washed hands before — yes - no

hand sanitizer before — yes - no

mask on you — yes - no

body temperature

air circulation — outdoors or inside

number of people

washed hands after — yes - no

hand sanitizer after — yes - no

PLACE and address   **DATE:**

your health:

NAMES include people you traveled with   **mask yes / no**

___

___

___

___

describe the social distancing

ARRIVAL TIME   AM / PM

DEPARTURE TIME   AM / PM

transportation

washed hands before   yes - no

hand sanitizer before   yes - no

mask on you   yes - no

body temperature

air circulation   outdoors or inside

number of people

washed hands after   yes - no

hand sanitizer after   yes - no

PLACE and address

DATE:

your health:

NAMES include people you traveled with

mask yes / no

___

___

___

___

describe the social distancing

ARRIVAL TIME AM / PM

DEPARTURE TIME AM / PM

transportation

washed hands before   yes - no

hand sanitizer before   yes - no

mask on you   yes - no

body temperature

air circulation   outdoors or inside

number of people

washed hands after   yes - no

hand sanitizer after   yes - no

PLACE and address

DATE:

your health:

NAMES include people you traveled with

mask yes / no

———

———

———

———

describe the social distancing

ARRIVAL TIME AM / PM

DEPARTURE TIME AM / PM

transportation

washed hands before — yes - no

hand sanitizer before — yes - no

mask on you — yes - no

body temperature

air circulation — outdoors or inside

number of people

washed hands after — yes - no

hand sanitizer after — yes - no

PLACE   and address   **DATE:**

your health:

NAMES   include people you traveled with   **mask yes / no**

___

___

___

___

describe the social distancing

ARRIVAL TIME   AM / PM

DEPARTURE TIME   AM / PM

transportation

washed hands before   yes - no

hand sanitizer before   yes - no

mask on you   yes - no

body temperature

air circulation   outdoors or inside

number of people

washed hands after   yes - no

hand sanitizer after   yes - no

PLACE and address

DATE:

your health:

NAMES include people you traveled with

mask yes / no

—

—

—

—

describe the social distancing

ARRIVAL TIME   AM / PM

DEPARTURE TIME   AM / PM

transportation

washed hands before yes - no

hand sanitizer before yes - no

mask on you yes - no

body temperature

air circulation outdoors or inside

number of people

washed hands after yes - no

hand sanitizer after yes - no

PLACE and address   DATE:

your health:

NAMES include people you traveled with   **mask yes / no**

___

___

___

___

describe the social distancing

ARRIVAL TIME   AM / PM

DEPARTURE TIME   AM / PM

transportation

washed hands before   yes - no

hand sanitizer before   yes - no

mask on you   yes - no

body temperature

air circulation   outdoors or inside

number of people

washed hands after   yes - no

hand sanitizer after   yes - no

PLACE and address   DATE:

your health:

NAMES include people you traveled with   **mask yes / no**

___

___

___

___

describe the social distancing

ARRIVAL TIME   AM / PM

DEPARTURE TIME   AM / PM

transportation

washed hands before   yes - no

hand sanitizer before   yes - no

mask on you   yes - no

body temperature

air circulation   outdoors or inside

number of people

washed hands after   yes - no

hand sanitizer after   yes - no

PLACE and address

DATE:

your health:

NAMES include people you traveled with

mask yes / no

___

___

___

___

describe the social distancing

ARRIVAL TIME AM / PM

DEPARTURE TIME AM / PM

transportation

washed hands before | yes - no

hand sanitizer before | yes - no

mask on you | yes - no

body temperature

air circulation | outdoors or inside

number of people

washed hands after | yes - no

hand sanitizer after | yes - no

PLACE   and address   **DATE:**

your health:

NAMES   include people you traveled with   **mask yes / no**

___

___

___

___

describe the social distancing

ARRIVAL TIME	AM / PM
DEPARTURE TIME	AM / PM
transportation	
washed hands before	yes - no
hand sanitizer before	yes - no
mask on you	yes - no
body temperature	
air circulation	outdoors or inside
number of people	
washed hands after	yes - no
hand sanitizer after	yes - no

PLACE and address   DATE:

your health:

NAMES include people you traveled with   **mask yes / no**

___

___

___

___

describe the social distancing

| **ARRIVAL TIME** | AM / PM |

| **DEPARTURE TIME** | AM / PM |

| transportation | |

| washed hands before | yes - no |

| hand sanitizer before | yes - no |

| mask on you | yes - no |

| body temperature | |

| air circulation | outdoors or inside |

| number of people | |

| washed hands after | yes - no |

| hand sanitizer after | yes - no |

PLACE and address

DATE:

your health:

NAMES include people you traveled with

mask yes / no

—

—

—

—

describe the social distancing

ARRIVAL TIME	AM / PM
DEPARTURE TIME	AM / PM
transportation	
washed hands before	yes - no
hand sanitizer before	yes - no
mask on you	yes - no
body temperature	
air circulation	outdoors or inside
number of people	
washed hands after	yes - no
hand sanitizer after	yes - no

PLACE and address

DATE:

your health:

NAMES include people you traveled with

mask yes / no

—

—

—

—

describe the social distancing

ARRIVAL TIME AM / PM

DEPARTURE TIME AM / PM

transportation

washed hands before | yes - no

hand sanitizer before | yes - no

mask on you | yes - no

body temperature

air circulation | outdoors or inside

number of people

washed hands after | yes - no

hand sanitizer after | yes - no

PLACE and address   DATE:

your health:

NAMES include people you traveled with   **mask yes / no**

___

___

___

___

describe the social distancing

ARRIVAL TIME   AM / PM

DEPARTURE TIME   AM / PM

transportation

washed hands before   yes - no

hand sanitizer before   yes - no

mask on you   yes - no

body temperature

air circulation   outdoors or inside

number of people

washed hands after   yes - no

hand sanitizer after   yes - no

PLACE and address   DATE:

your health:

NAMES include people you traveled with   mask yes / no

___

___

___

___

describe the social distancing

ARRIVAL TIME   AM / PM

DEPARTURE TIME   AM / PM

transportation

washed hands before   yes - no

hand sanitizer before   yes - no

mask on you   yes - no

body temperature

air circulation   outdoors or inside

number of people

washed hands after   yes - no

hand sanitizer after   yes - no

PLACE and address

DATE:

your health:

NAMES include people you traveled with

mask yes / no

___

___

___

___

describe the social distancing

ARRIVAL TIME AM / PM

DEPARTURE TIME AM / PM

transportation

washed hands before   yes - no

hand sanitizer before   yes - no

mask on you   yes - no

body temperature

air circulation   outdoors or inside

number of people

washed hands after   yes - no

hand sanitizer after   yes - no

PLACE and address   **DATE:**

your health:

NAMES include people you traveled with   **mask yes / no**

—

—

—

—

describe the social distancing

ARRIVAL TIME   AM / PM

DEPARTURE TIME   AM / PM

transportation

washed hands before   yes - no

hand sanitizer before   yes - no

mask on you   yes - no

body temperature

air circulation   outdoors or inside

number of people

washed hands after   yes - no

hand sanitizer after   yes - no

PLACE and address

DATE:

your health:

NAMES include people you traveled with

mask yes / no

___

___

___

___

describe the social distancing

ARRIVAL TIME   AM / PM

DEPARTURE TIME   AM / PM

transportation

washed hands before   yes - no

hand sanitizer before   yes - no

mask on you   yes - no

body temperature

air circulation   outdoors or inside

number of people

washed hands after   yes - no

hand sanitizer after   yes - no

PLACE and address

DATE:

your health:

NAMES include people you traveled with

mask yes / no

____

____

____

____

describe the social distancing

ARRIVAL TIME AM / PM

DEPARTURE TIME AM / PM

transportation

washed hands before — yes - no

hand sanitizer before — yes - no

mask on you — yes - no

body temperature

air circulation — outdoors or inside

number of people

washed hands after — yes - no

hand sanitizer after — yes - no

PLACE and address   DATE:

your health:

NAMES include people you traveled with   **mask yes / no**

—

—

—

—

describe the social distancing

ARRIVAL TIME   AM / PM

DEPARTURE TIME   AM / PM

transportation

washed hands before   yes - no

hand sanitizer before   yes - no

mask on you   yes - no

body temperature

air circulation   outdoors or inside

number of people

washed hands after   yes - no

hand sanitizer after   yes - no

PLACE and address   DATE:

your health:

NAMES include people you traveled with   **mask yes / no**

___

___

___

___

describe the social distancing

ARRIVAL TIME 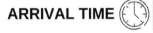   AM / PM

DEPARTURE TIME 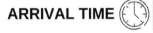   AM / PM

transportation

washed hands before   yes - no

hand sanitizer before   yes - no

mask on you   yes - no

body temperature

air circulation   outdoors or inside

number of people

washed hands after   yes - no

hand sanitizer after   yes - no

PLACE and address

DATE:

your health:

NAMES include people you traveled with

mask yes / no

———

———

———

———

describe the social distancing

ARRIVAL TIME AM / PM

DEPARTURE TIME AM / PM

transportation

washed hands before   yes - no

hand sanitizer before   yes - no

mask on you   yes - no

body temperature

air circulation   outdoors or inside

number of people

washed hands after   yes - no

hand sanitizer after   yes - no

PLACE and address   **DATE:**

your health:

NAMES include people you traveled with   **mask yes / no**

‗

‗

‗

‗

describe the social distancing

ARRIVAL TIME   AM / PM

DEPARTURE TIME   AM / PM

transportation

washed hands before   yes - no

hand sanitizer before   yes - no

mask on you   yes - no

body temperature

air circulation   outdoors or inside

number of people

washed hands after   yes - no

hand sanitizer after   yes - no

PLACE and address

DATE:

your health:

NAMES include people you traveled with

mask yes / no

___

___

___

___

describe the social distancing

ARRIVAL TIME   AM / PM

DEPARTURE TIME   AM / PM

transportation

washed hands before   yes - no

hand sanitizer before   yes - no

mask on you   yes - no

body temperature

air circulation   outdoors or inside

number of people

washed hands after   yes - no

hand sanitizer after   yes - no

PLACE and address   DATE:

your health:

NAMES include people you traveled with   **mask yes / no**

___

___

___

___

describe the social distancing

ARRIVAL TIME   AM / PM

DEPARTURE TIME   AM / PM

transportation

washed hands before   yes - no

hand sanitizer before   yes - no

mask on you   yes - no

body temperature

air circulation   outdoors or inside

number of people

washed hands after   yes - no

hand sanitizer after   yes - no

PLACE and address   DATE:

your health:

NAMES include people you traveled with   **mask yes / no**

___

___

___

___

describe the social distancing

ARRIVAL TIME   AM / PM

DEPARTURE TIME   AM / PM

transportation

washed hands before   yes - no

hand sanitizer before   yes - no

mask on you   yes - no

body temperature

air circulation   outdoors or inside

number of people

washed hands after   yes - no

hand sanitizer after   yes - no

PLACE and address

DATE:

your health:

NAMES include people you traveled with

mask yes / no

___

___

___

___

describe the social distancing

ARRIVAL TIME   AM / PM

DEPARTURE TIME   AM / PM

transportation

washed hands before   yes - no

hand sanitizer before   yes - no

mask on you   yes - no

body temperature

air circulation   outdoors or inside

number of people

washed hands after   yes - no

hand sanitizer after   yes - no

PLACE and address   **DATE:**

your health:

NAMES include people you traveled with   **mask yes / no**

___

___

___

___

describe the social distancing

ARRIVAL TIME		AM / PM
DEPARTURE TIME		AM / PM
transportation		
washed hands before		yes - no
hand sanitizer before		yes - no
mask on you		yes - no
body temperature		
air circulation		outdoors or inside
number of people		
washed hands after		yes - no
hand sanitizer after		yes - no

PLACE and address

DATE:

your health:

NAMES include people you traveled with

mask yes / no

___

___

___

___

describe the social distancing

ARRIVAL TIME   AM / PM

DEPARTURE TIME   AM / PM

transportation

washed hands before yes - no

hand sanitizer before yes - no

mask on you yes - no

body temperature

air circulation outdoors or inside

number of people

washed hands after yes - no

hand sanitizer after yes - no

PLACE and address   **DATE:**

your health:

NAMES include people you traveled with   **mask yes / no**

___

___

___

___

describe the social distancing

ARRIVAL TIME   AM / PM

DEPARTURE TIME   AM / PM

transportation

washed hands before   yes - no

hand sanitizer before   yes - no

mask on you   yes - no

body temperature

air circulation   outdoors or inside

number of people

washed hands after   yes - no

hand sanitizer after   yes - no

PLACE and address

DATE:

your health:

NAMES include people you traveled with

mask yes / no

——

——

——

——

describe the social distancing

ARRIVAL TIME AM / PM

DEPARTURE TIME AM / PM

transportation

washed hands before   yes - no

hand sanitizer before   yes - no

mask on you   yes - no

body temperature

air circulation   outdoors or inside

number of people

washed hands after   yes - no

hand sanitizer after   yes - no

PLACE and address

DATE:

your health:

NAMES include people you traveled with

mask yes / no

___

___

___

___

describe the social distancing

ARRIVAL TIME   AM / PM

DEPARTURE TIME   AM / PM

transportation

washed hands before   yes - no

hand sanitizer before   yes - no

mask on you   yes - no

body temperature

air circulation   outdoors or inside

number of people

washed hands after   yes - no

hand sanitizer after   yes - no

PLACE and address   DATE:

your health:

NAMES include people you traveled with   **mask yes / no**

____

____

____

____

describe the social distancing

ARRIVAL TIME 🕐	AM / PM
DEPARTURE TIME 🕐	AM / PM
transportation 🚶 🚴 🚗	
washed hands before	yes - no
hand sanitizer before	yes - no
mask on you	yes - no
body temperature	
air circulation	outdoors or inside
number of people	
washed hands after	yes - no
hand sanitizer after	yes - no

PLACE and address

DATE:

your health:

NAMES include people you traveled with

mask yes / no

___

___

___

___

describe the social distancing

ARRIVAL TIME   AM / PM

DEPARTURE TIME   AM / PM

transportation

washed hands before   yes - no

hand sanitizer before   yes - no

mask on you   yes - no

body temperature

air circulation   outdoors or inside

number of people

washed hands after   yes - no

hand sanitizer after   yes - no

PLACE   and address   DATE:

your health:

NAMES   include people you traveled with   **mask yes / no**

describe the social distancing

ARRIVAL TIME   AM / PM

DEPARTURE TIME   AM / PM

transportation

washed hands before   yes - no

hand sanitizer before   yes - no

mask on you   yes - no

body temperature

air circulation   outdoors or inside

number of people

washed hands after   yes - no

hand sanitizer after   yes - no

PLACE and address   DATE:

your health:

NAMES include people you traveled with   **mask yes / no**

___

___

___

___

describe the social distancing

ARRIVAL TIME 🕐	AM / PM
DEPARTURE TIME 🕐	AM / PM
transportation 🚶 🚴 🚗	
washed hands before	yes - no
hand sanitizer before	yes - no
mask on you	yes - no
body temperature	
air circulation	outdoors or inside
number of people	
washed hands after	yes - no
hand sanitizer after	yes - no

PLACE   and address   DATE:

your health:

NAMES   include people you traveled with   **mask yes / no**

___

___

___

___

describe the social distancing

ARRIVAL TIME   AM / PM

DEPARTURE TIME   AM / PM

transportation

washed hands before   yes - no

hand sanitizer before   yes - no

mask on you   yes - no

body temperature

air circulation   outdoors or inside

number of people

washed hands after   yes - no

hand sanitizer after   yes - no

PLACE and address

DATE:

your health:

NAMES include people you traveled with

mask yes / no

___

___

___

___

describe the social distancing

ARRIVAL TIME 🕐 AM / PM

DEPARTURE TIME 🕐 AM / PM

transportation

washed hands before — yes - no

hand sanitizer before — yes - no

mask on you — yes - no

body temperature

air circulation — outdoors or inside

number of people

washed hands after — yes - no

hand sanitizer after — yes - no

PLACE and address

DATE:

your health:

NAMES include people you traveled with

mask yes / no

___

___

___

___

describe the social distancing

ARRIVAL TIME AM / PM

DEPARTURE TIME AM / PM

transportation

washed hands before | yes - no

hand sanitizer before | yes - no

mask on you | yes - no

body temperature

air circulation | outdoors or inside

number of people

washed hands after | yes - no

hand sanitizer after | yes - no

PLACE and address   DATE:

your health:

NAMES include people you traveled with   **mask yes / no**

___

___

___

___

describe the social distancing

ARRIVAL TIME 🕐   AM / PM

DEPARTURE TIME 🕐   AM / PM

transportation

washed hands before   yes - no

hand sanitizer before   yes - no

mask on you   yes - no

body temperature

air circulation   outdoors or inside

number of people

washed hands after   yes - no

hand sanitizer after   yes - no

PLACE and address

DATE:

your health:

NAMES include people you traveled with

mask yes / no

—

—

—

—

describe the social distancing

ARRIVAL TIME   AM / PM

DEPARTURE TIME   AM / PM

transportation

washed hands before   yes - no

hand sanitizer before   yes - no

mask on you   yes - no

body temperature

air circulation   outdoors or inside

number of people

washed hands after   yes - no

hand sanitizer after   yes - no

PLACE and address

DATE:

your health:

NAMES include people you traveled with

mask yes / no

___

___

___

___

describe the social distancing

ARRIVAL TIME 🕐   AM / PM

DEPARTURE TIME 🕐   AM / PM

transportation 🚶 🚴 🚗

washed hands before	yes - no
hand sanitizer before	yes - no
mask on you	yes - no
body temperature	
air circulation	outdoors or inside
number of people	
washed hands after	yes - no
hand sanitizer after	yes - no

PLACE and address   DATE:

your health:

NAMES include people you traveled with   mask yes / no

___

___

___

___

describe the social distancing

ARRIVAL TIME   AM / PM

DEPARTURE TIME   AM / PM

transportation

washed hands before   yes - no

hand sanitizer before   yes - no

mask on you   yes - no

body temperature

air circulation   outdoors or inside

number of people

washed hands after   yes - no

hand sanitizer after   yes - no

PLACE and address   DATE:

your health:

NAMES include people you traveled with   **mask yes / no**

___

___

___

___

describe the social distancing

ARRIVAL TIME   AM / PM

DEPARTURE TIME   AM / PM

transportation

washed hands before   yes - no

hand sanitizer before   yes - no

mask on you   yes - no

body temperature

air circulation   outdoors or inside

number of people

washed hands after   yes - no

hand sanitizer after   yes - no

PLACE and address   DATE:

your health:

NAMES include people you traveled with   mask yes / no

___

___

___

___

describe the social distancing

ARRIVAL TIME   AM / PM

DEPARTURE TIME   AM / PM

transportation

washed hands before   yes - no

hand sanitizer before   yes - no

mask on you   yes - no

body temperature

air circulation   outdoors or inside

number of people

washed hands after   yes - no

hand sanitizer after   yes - no

PLACE and address   DATE:

your health:

NAMES include people you traveled with   **mask yes / no**

___

___

___

___

describe the social distancing

ARRIVAL TIME   AM / PM

DEPARTURE TIME   AM / PM

transportation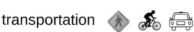

washed hands before   yes - no

hand sanitizer before   yes - no

mask on you   yes - no

body temperature

air circulation   outdoors or inside

number of people

washed hands after   yes - no

hand sanitizer after   yes - no

PLACE and address

DATE:

your health:

NAMES include people you traveled with

mask yes / no

___

___

___

___

describe the social distancing

ARRIVAL TIME 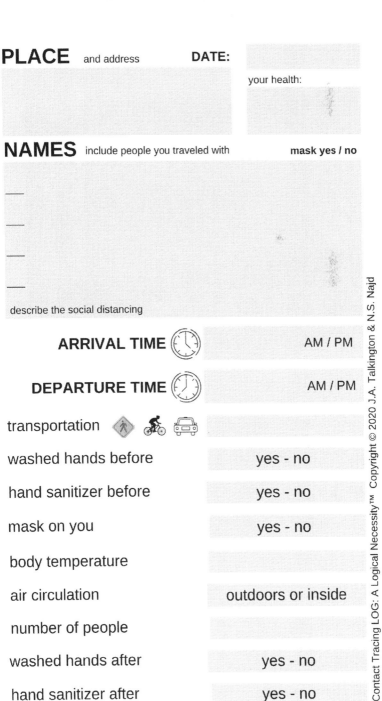 AM / PM

DEPARTURE TIME AM / PM

transportation

washed hands before yes - no

hand sanitizer before yes - no

mask on you yes - no

body temperature

air circulation outdoors or inside

number of people

washed hands after yes - no

hand sanitizer after yes - no

PLACE and address   DATE:

your health:

NAMES include people you traveled with   **mask yes / no**

___

___

___

___

describe the social distancing

ARRIVAL TIME 🕐   AM / PM

DEPARTURE TIME 🕐   AM / PM

transportation

washed hands before   yes - no

hand sanitizer before   yes - no

mask on you   yes - no

body temperature

air circulation   outdoors or inside

number of people

washed hands after   yes - no

hand sanitizer after   yes - no

PLACE and address   DATE:

your health:

NAMES include people you traveled with   **mask yes / no**

____

____

____

____

describe the social distancing

ARRIVAL TIME   AM / PM

DEPARTURE TIME   AM / PM

transportation

washed hands before   yes - no

hand sanitizer before   yes - no

mask on you   yes - no

body temperature

air circulation   outdoors or inside

number of people

washed hands after   yes - no

hand sanitizer after   yes - no

PLACE and address

DATE:

your health:

NAMES include people you traveled with

mask yes / no

___

___

___

___

describe the social distancing

ARRIVAL TIME AM / PM

DEPARTURE TIME AM / PM

transportation

washed hands before | yes - no

hand sanitizer before | yes - no

mask on you | yes - no

body temperature

air circulation | outdoors or inside

number of people

washed hands after | yes - no

hand sanitizer after | yes - no

PLACE and address

DATE:

your health:

NAMES include people you traveled with

mask yes / no

——

——

——

——

describe the social distancing

ARRIVAL TIME AM / PM

DEPARTURE TIME AM / PM

transportation

washed hands before   yes - no

hand sanitizer before   yes - no

mask on you   yes - no

body temperature

air circulation   outdoors or inside

number of people

washed hands after   yes - no

hand sanitizer after   yes - no

PLACE and address

DATE:

your health:

NAMES include people you traveled with

mask yes / no

____

____

____

____

describe the social distancing

ARRIVAL TIME AM / PM

DEPARTURE TIME AM / PM

transportation

washed hands before — yes - no

hand sanitizer before — yes - no

mask on you — yes - no

body temperature

air circulation — outdoors or inside

number of people

washed hands after — yes - no

hand sanitizer after — yes - no

Contact Tracing LOG: A Logical Necessity™ Copyright © 2020 J.A. Talkington & N.S. Najd

PLACE and address

DATE:

your health:

NAMES include people you traveled with

mask yes / no

___

___

___

___

describe the social distancing

ARRIVAL TIME   AM / PM

DEPARTURE TIME   AM / PM

transportation

washed hands before   yes - no

hand sanitizer before   yes - no

mask on you   yes - no

body temperature

air circulation   outdoors or inside

number of people

washed hands after   yes - no

hand sanitizer after   yes - no

PLACE and address   DATE:

your health:

NAMES include people you traveled with   **mask yes / no**

___

___

___

___

describe the social distancing

ARRIVAL TIME 🕐		AM / PM
DEPARTURE TIME 🕐		AM / PM
transportation		
washed hands before	yes - no	
hand sanitizer before	yes - no	
mask on you	yes - no	
body temperature		
air circulation	outdoors or inside	
number of people		
washed hands after	yes - no	
hand sanitizer after	yes - no	

PLACE and address　　　　DATE:

your health:

NAMES include people you traveled with　　　mask yes / no

—

—

—

—

describe the social distancing

ARRIVAL TIME 　　　AM / PM

DEPARTURE TIME 　　　AM / PM

transportation

washed hands before　　　yes - no

hand sanitizer before　　　yes - no

mask on you　　　yes - no

body temperature

air circulation　　　outdoors or inside

number of people

washed hands after　　　yes - no

hand sanitizer after　　　yes - no

PLACE and address DATE:

your health:

NAMES include people you traveled with

mask yes / no

___

___

___

___

describe the social distancing

ARRIVAL TIME 🕐 AM / PM

DEPARTURE TIME 🕐 AM / PM

transportation

washed hands before — yes - no

hand sanitizer before — yes - no

mask on you — yes - no

body temperature

air circulation — outdoors or inside

number of people

washed hands after — yes - no

hand sanitizer after — yes - no

PLACE and address

DATE:

your health:

NAMES include people you traveled with

mask yes / no

___

___

___

___

describe the social distancing

ARRIVAL TIME   AM / PM

DEPARTURE TIME   AM / PM

transportation

washed hands before   yes - no

hand sanitizer before   yes - no

mask on you   yes - no

body temperature

air circulation   outdoors or inside

number of people

washed hands after   yes - no

hand sanitizer after   yes - no

PLACE and address   DATE:

your health:

NAMES include people you traveled with   **mask yes / no**

___

___

___

___

describe the social distancing

ARRIVAL TIME 🕐   AM / PM

DEPARTURE TIME 🕐   AM / PM

transportation 🚶 🚴 🚗

washed hands before   yes - no

hand sanitizer before   yes - no

mask on you   yes - no

body temperature

air circulation   outdoors or inside

number of people

washed hands after   yes - no

hand sanitizer after   yes - no

PLACE and address   DATE:

your health:

NAMES include people you traveled with   **mask yes / no**

___

___

___

___

describe the social distancing

ARRIVAL TIME   AM / PM

DEPARTURE TIME   AM / PM

transportation

washed hands before   yes - no

hand sanitizer before   yes - no

mask on you   yes - no

body temperature

air circulation   outdoors or inside

number of people

washed hands after   yes - no

hand sanitizer after   yes - no

PLACE and address

DATE:

your health:

NAMES include people you traveled with

mask yes / no

___

___

___

___

describe the social distancing

ARRIVAL TIME 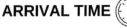 AM / PM

DEPARTURE TIME AM / PM

transportation

washed hands before | yes - no

hand sanitizer before | yes - no

mask on you | yes - no

body temperature

air circulation | outdoors or inside

number of people

washed hands after | yes - no

hand sanitizer after | yes - no

PLACE and address   DATE:

your health:

NAMES include people you traveled with   mask yes / no

____

____

____

____

describe the social distancing

ARRIVAL TIME   AM / PM

DEPARTURE TIME   AM / PM

transportation

washed hands before   yes - no

hand sanitizer before   yes - no

mask on you   yes - no

body temperature

air circulation   outdoors or inside

number of people

washed hands after   yes - no

hand sanitizer after   yes - no

PLACE and address

DATE:

your health:

NAMES include people you traveled with

mask yes / no

___

___

___

___

describe the social distancing

ARRIVAL TIME   AM / PM

DEPARTURE TIME   AM / PM

transportation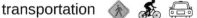

washed hands before yes - no

hand sanitizer before yes - no

mask on you yes - no

body temperature

air circulation outdoors or inside

number of people

washed hands after yes - no

hand sanitizer after yes - no

PLACE and address   **DATE:**

your health:

NAMES include people you traveled with   **mask yes / no**

___

___

___

___

describe the social distancing

ARRIVAL TIME   AM / PM

DEPARTURE TIME   AM / PM

transportation

washed hands before   yes - no

hand sanitizer before   yes - no

mask on you   yes - no

body temperature

air circulation   outdoors or inside

number of people

washed hands after   yes - no

hand sanitizer after   yes - no

PLACE and address

DATE:

your health:

NAMES include people you traveled with

mask yes / no

____

____

____

____

describe the social distancing

ARRIVAL TIME	AM / PM
DEPARTURE TIME	AM / PM
transportation	
washed hands before	yes - no
hand sanitizer before	yes - no
mask on you	yes - no
body temperature	
air circulation	outdoors or inside
number of people	
washed hands after	yes - no
hand sanitizer after	yes - no

PLACE and address   DATE:

your health:

NAMES include people you traveled with   **mask yes / no**

___

___

___

___

describe the social distancing

ARRIVAL TIME   AM / PM

DEPARTURE TIME   AM / PM

transportation

washed hands before   yes - no

hand sanitizer before   yes - no

mask on you   yes - no

body temperature

air circulation   outdoors or inside

number of people

washed hands after   yes - no

hand sanitizer after   yes - no

PLACE and address

DATE:

your health:

NAMES include people you traveled with

mask yes / no

___

___

___

___

describe the social distancing

ARRIVAL TIME AM / PM

DEPARTURE TIME AM / PM

transportation

washed hands before   yes - no

hand sanitizer before   yes - no

mask on you   yes - no

body temperature

air circulation   outdoors or inside

number of people

washed hands after   yes - no

hand sanitizer after   yes - no

PLACE and address

DATE:

your health:

NAMES include people you traveled with

mask yes / no

___

___

___

___

describe the social distancing

ARRIVAL TIME AM / PM

DEPARTURE TIME AM / PM

transportation

washed hands before | yes - no

hand sanitizer before | yes - no

mask on you | yes - no

body temperature

air circulation | outdoors or inside

number of people

washed hands after | yes - no

hand sanitizer after | yes - no

PLACE and address

DATE:

your health:

NAMES include people you traveled with

mask yes / no

___

___

___

___

describe the social distancing

ARRIVAL TIME   AM / PM

DEPARTURE TIME   AM / PM

transportation

washed hands before   yes - no

hand sanitizer before   yes - no

mask on you   yes - no

body temperature

air circulation   outdoors or inside

number of people

washed hands after   yes - no

hand sanitizer after   yes - no

PLACE and address

DATE:

your health:

NAMES include people you traveled with

mask yes / no

___

___

___

___

describe the social distancing

ARRIVAL TIME   AM / PM

DEPARTURE TIME   AM / PM

transportation

washed hands before   yes - no

hand sanitizer before   yes - no

mask on you   yes - no

body temperature

air circulation   outdoors or inside

number of people

washed hands after   yes - no

hand sanitizer after   yes - no

PLACE and address   DATE:

your health:

NAMES include people you traveled with   **mask yes / no**

___

___

___

___

describe the social distancing

ARRIVAL TIME 🕐	AM / PM
DEPARTURE TIME 🕐	AM / PM
transportation	
washed hands before	yes - no
hand sanitizer before	yes - no
mask on you	yes - no
body temperature	
air circulation	outdoors or inside
number of people	
washed hands after	yes - no
hand sanitizer after	yes - no

PLACE and address   DATE:

your health:

NAMES include people you traveled with   **mask yes / no**

___

___

___

___

describe the social distancing

ARRIVAL TIME   AM / PM

DEPARTURE TIME   AM / PM

transportation

washed hands before   yes - no

hand sanitizer before   yes - no

mask on you   yes - no

body temperature

air circulation   outdoors or inside

number of people

washed hands after   yes - no

hand sanitizer after   yes - no

PLACE and address

DATE:

your health:

NAMES include people you traveled with

mask yes / no

____

____

____

____

describe the social distancing

ARRIVAL TIME AM / PM

DEPARTURE TIME AM / PM

transportation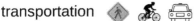

washed hands before | yes - no

hand sanitizer before | yes - no

mask on you | yes - no

body temperature

air circulation | outdoors or inside

number of people

washed hands after | yes - no

hand sanitizer after | yes - no

PLACE and address   DATE:

your health:

NAMES include people you traveled with   mask yes / no

___

___

___

___

describe the social distancing

ARRIVAL TIME   AM / PM

DEPARTURE TIME   AM / PM

transportation

washed hands before   yes - no

hand sanitizer before   yes - no

mask on you   yes - no

body temperature

air circulation   outdoors or inside

number of people

washed hands after   yes - no

hand sanitizer after   yes - no

PLACE   and address   DATE:

your health:

NAMES   include people you traveled with   **mask yes / no**

___

___

___

___

describe the social distancing

ARRIVAL TIME   AM / PM

DEPARTURE TIME   AM / PM

transportation

washed hands before   yes - no

hand sanitizer before   yes - no

mask on you   yes - no

body temperature

air circulation   outdoors or inside

number of people

washed hands after   yes - no

hand sanitizer after   yes - no

PLACE and address

DATE:

your health:

NAMES include people you traveled with

mask yes / no

____

____

____

____

describe the social distancing

ARRIVAL TIME   AM / PM

DEPARTURE TIME   AM / PM

transportation

washed hands before   yes - no

hand sanitizer before   yes - no

mask on you   yes - no

body temperature

air circulation   outdoors or inside

number of people

washed hands after   yes - no

hand sanitizer after   yes - no

PLACE and address
DATE:

your health:

NAMES include people you traveled with

mask yes / no

___

___

___

___

describe the social distancing

ARRIVAL TIME AM / PM

DEPARTURE TIME AM / PM

transportation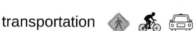

washed hands before | yes - no

hand sanitizer before | yes - no

mask on you | yes - no

body temperature

air circulation | outdoors or inside

number of people

washed hands after | yes - no

hand sanitizer after | yes - no

PLACE and address

DATE:

your health:

NAMES include people you traveled with

mask yes / no

___

___

___

___

describe the social distancing

ARRIVAL TIME   AM / PM

DEPARTURE TIME   AM / PM

transportation

washed hands before   yes - no

hand sanitizer before   yes - no

mask on you   yes - no

body temperature

air circulation   outdoors or inside

number of people

washed hands after   yes - no

hand sanitizer after   yes - no

PLACE and address

DATE:

your health:

NAMES include people you traveled with

mask yes / no

___

___

___

___

describe the social distancing

ARRIVAL TIME	AM / PM
DEPARTURE TIME	AM / PM
transportation 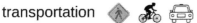	
washed hands before	yes - no
hand sanitizer before	yes - no
mask on you	yes - no
body temperature	
air circulation	outdoors or inside
number of people	
washed hands after	yes - no
hand sanitizer after	yes - no

PLACE and address   DATE:

your health:

NAMES include people you traveled with   mask yes / no

___

___

___

___

describe the social distancing

ARRIVAL TIME		AM / PM
DEPARTURE TIME		AM / PM
transportation		
washed hands before		yes - no
hand sanitizer before		yes - no
mask on you		yes - no
body temperature		
air circulation		outdoors or inside
number of people		
washed hands after		yes - no
hand sanitizer after		yes - no

PLACE and address   DATE:

your health:

NAMES include people you traveled with   mask yes / no

___

___

___

___

describe the social distancing

ARRIVAL TIME   AM / PM

DEPARTURE TIME   AM / PM

transportation

washed hands before   yes - no

hand sanitizer before   yes - no

mask on you   yes - no

body temperature

air circulation   outdoors or inside

number of people

washed hands after   yes - no

hand sanitizer after   yes - no

PLACE and address   DATE:

your health:

NAMES include people you traveled with   **mask yes / no**

___

___

___

___

describe the social distancing

ARRIVAL TIME   AM / PM

DEPARTURE TIME   AM / PM

transportation

washed hands before   yes - no

hand sanitizer before   yes - no

mask on you   yes - no

body temperature

air circulation   outdoors or inside

number of people

washed hands after   yes - no

hand sanitizer after   yes - no

PLACE and address   DATE:

your health:

NAMES include people you traveled with   **mask yes / no**

___

___

___

___

describe the social distancing

ARRIVAL TIME   AM / PM

DEPARTURE TIME   AM / PM

transportation

washed hands before   yes - no

hand sanitizer before   yes - no

mask on you   yes - no

body temperature

air circulation   outdoors or inside

number of people

washed hands after   yes - no

hand sanitizer after   yes - no

PLACE and address

DATE:

your health:

NAMES include people you traveled with

mask yes / no

___

___

___

___

describe the social distancing

ARRIVAL TIME   AM / PM

DEPARTURE TIME   AM / PM

transportation

washed hands before   yes - no

hand sanitizer before   yes - no

mask on you   yes - no

body temperature

air circulation   outdoors or inside

number of people

washed hands after   yes - no

hand sanitizer after   yes - no

PLACE and address

DATE:

your health:

NAMES include people you traveled with

mask yes / no

___

___

___

___

describe the social distancing

ARRIVAL TIME 🕐 AM / PM

DEPARTURE TIME 🕐 AM / PM

transportation

washed hands before — yes - no

hand sanitizer before — yes - no

mask on you — yes - no

body temperature

air circulation — outdoors or inside

number of people

washed hands after — yes - no

hand sanitizer after — yes - no

PLACE and address

DATE:

your health:

NAMES include people you traveled with

mask yes / no

___

___

___

___

describe the social distancing

ARRIVAL TIME 　　　　AM / PM

DEPARTURE TIME 　　　AM / PM

transportation

washed hands before　　　yes - no

hand sanitizer before　　　yes - no

mask on you　　　yes - no

body temperature

air circulation　　　outdoors or inside

number of people

washed hands after　　　yes - no

hand sanitizer after　　　yes - no

PLACE and address

DATE:

your health:

NAMES include people you traveled with

mask yes / no

____

____

____

____

describe the social distancing

ARRIVAL TIME AM / PM

DEPARTURE TIME AM / PM

transportation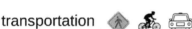

washed hands before — yes - no

hand sanitizer before — yes - no

mask on you — yes - no

body temperature

air circulation — outdoors or inside

number of people

washed hands after — yes - no

hand sanitizer after — yes - no

PLACE and address

DATE:

your health:

NAMES include people you traveled with

mask yes / no

___

___

___

___

describe the social distancing

ARRIVAL TIME   AM / PM

DEPARTURE TIME   AM / PM

transportation

washed hands before   yes - no

hand sanitizer before   yes - no

mask on you   yes - no

body temperature

air circulation   outdoors or inside

number of people

washed hands after   yes - no

hand sanitizer after   yes - no

PLACE and address

DATE:

your health:

NAMES include people you traveled with

mask yes / no

___

___

___

___

describe the social distancing

ARRIVAL TIME 🕐		AM / PM
DEPARTURE TIME 🕐		AM / PM
transportation 🚶 🚴 🚗		
washed hands before		yes - no
hand sanitizer before		yes - no
mask on you		yes - no
body temperature		
air circulation		outdoors or inside
number of people		
washed hands after		yes - no
hand sanitizer after		yes - no

PLACE and address

DATE:

your health:

NAMES include people you traveled with

mask yes / no

___

___

___

___

describe the social distancing

ARRIVAL TIME   AM / PM

DEPARTURE TIME   AM / PM

transportation

washed hands before   yes - no

hand sanitizer before   yes - no

mask on you   yes - no

body temperature

air circulation   outdoors or inside

number of people

washed hands after   yes - no

hand sanitizer after   yes - no

PLACE and address   DATE:

your health:

NAMES include people you traveled with   **mask yes / no**

___

___

___

___

describe the social distancing

ARRIVAL TIME   AM / PM

DEPARTURE TIME   AM / PM

transportation

washed hands before   yes - no

hand sanitizer before   yes - no

mask on you   yes - no

body temperature

air circulation   outdoors or inside

number of people

washed hands after   yes - no

hand sanitizer after   yes - no

PLACE and address   DATE:

your health:

NAMES include people you traveled with   **mask yes / no**

___

___

___

___

describe the social distancing

ARRIVAL TIME   AM / PM

DEPARTURE TIME   AM / PM

transportation

washed hands before   yes - no

hand sanitizer before   yes - no

mask on you   yes - no

body temperature

air circulation   outdoors or inside

number of people

washed hands after   yes - no

hand sanitizer after   yes - no

PLACE and address   DATE:

your health:

NAMES include people you traveled with

mask yes / no

___

___

___

___

describe the social distancing

ARRIVAL TIME 🕐   AM / PM

DEPARTURE TIME 🕐   AM / PM

transportation

washed hands before   yes - no

hand sanitizer before   yes - no

mask on you   yes - no

body temperature

air circulation   outdoors or inside

number of people

washed hands after   yes - no

hand sanitizer after   yes - no

Contact Tracing LOG: A Logical Necessity™ Copyright © 2020 J.A. Talkington & N.S. Najd

PLACE and address   DATE:

your health:

NAMES include people you traveled with   **mask yes / no**

____

____

____

____

describe the social distancing

ARRIVAL TIME   AM / PM

DEPARTURE TIME   AM / PM

transportation

washed hands before   yes - no

hand sanitizer before   yes - no

mask on you   yes - no

body temperature

air circulation   outdoors or inside

number of people

washed hands after   yes - no

hand sanitizer after   yes - no

PLACE and address

DATE:

your health:

NAMES include people you traveled with

mask yes / no

___

___

___

___

describe the social distancing

ARRIVAL TIME 🕐 AM / PM

DEPARTURE TIME 🕐 AM / PM

transportation 🚶 🚴 🚗

washed hands before	yes - no
hand sanitizer before	yes - no
mask on you	yes - no
body temperature	
air circulation	outdoors or inside
number of people	
washed hands after	yes - no
hand sanitizer after	yes - no

PLACE and address   DATE:

your health:

NAMES include people you traveled with   **mask yes / no**

___

___

___

___

describe the social distancing

ARRIVAL TIME   AM / PM

DEPARTURE TIME   AM / PM

transportation

washed hands before   yes - no

hand sanitizer before   yes - no

mask on you   yes - no

body temperature

air circulation   outdoors or inside

number of people

washed hands after   yes - no

hand sanitizer after   yes - no

PLACE and address

DATE:

your health:

NAMES include people you traveled with

mask yes / no

___

___

___

___

describe the social distancing

ARRIVAL TIME 🕐   AM / PM

DEPARTURE TIME 🕐   AM / PM

transportation

washed hands before   yes - no

hand sanitizer before   yes - no

mask on you   yes - no

body temperature

air circulation   outdoors or inside

number of people

washed hands after   yes - no

hand sanitizer after   yes - no

PLACE and address   DATE:

your health:

NAMES include people you traveled with   **mask yes / no**

___

___

___

___

describe the social distancing

ARRIVAL TIME   AM / PM

DEPARTURE TIME   AM / PM

transportation

washed hands before   yes - no

hand sanitizer before   yes - no

mask on you   yes - no

body temperature

air circulation   outdoors or inside

number of people

washed hands after   yes - no

hand sanitizer after   yes - no

PLACE and address

DATE:

your health:

NAMES include people you traveled with

mask yes / no

___

___

___

___

describe the social distancing

ARRIVAL TIME 🕐 AM / PM

DEPARTURE TIME 🕐 AM / PM

transportation

washed hands before   yes - no

hand sanitizer before   yes - no

mask on you   yes - no

body temperature

air circulation   outdoors or inside

number of people

washed hands after   yes - no

hand sanitizer after   yes - no

PLACE and address   DATE:

your health:

NAMES include people you traveled with   **mask yes / no**

———

———

———

———

describe the social distancing

ARRIVAL TIME   AM / PM

DEPARTURE TIME   AM / PM

transportation

washed hands before   yes - no

hand sanitizer before   yes - no

mask on you   yes - no

body temperature

air circulation   outdoors or inside

number of people

washed hands after   yes - no

hand sanitizer after   yes - no

PLACE and address   DATE:

your health:

NAMES include people you traveled with

mask yes / no

___

___

___

___

describe the social distancing

ARRIVAL TIME AM / PM

DEPARTURE TIME AM / PM

transportation

washed hands before   yes - no

hand sanitizer before   yes - no

mask on you   yes - no

body temperature

air circulation   outdoors or inside

number of people

washed hands after   yes - no

hand sanitizer after   yes - no

PLACE and address

DATE:

your health:

NAMES include people you traveled with

mask yes / no

___

___

___

___

describe the social distancing

ARRIVAL TIME 🕐   AM / PM

DEPARTURE TIME 🕐   AM / PM

transportation 🚶 🚴 🚗

washed hands before   yes - no

hand sanitizer before   yes - no

mask on you   yes - no

body temperature

air circulation   outdoors or inside

number of people

washed hands after   yes - no

hand sanitizer after   yes - no

PLACE and address   DATE:

your health:

NAMES include people you traveled with   **mask yes / no**

___

___

___

___

describe the social distancing

ARRIVAL TIME 🕐	AM / PM
DEPARTURE TIME 🕐	AM / PM
transportation	
washed hands before	yes - no
hand sanitizer before	yes - no
mask on you	yes - no
body temperature	
air circulation	outdoors or inside
number of people	
washed hands after	yes - no
hand sanitizer after	yes - no

PLACE and address   DATE:

your health:

NAMES include people you traveled with   **mask yes / no**

___

___

___

___

describe the social distancing

ARRIVAL TIME 🕐   AM / PM

DEPARTURE TIME 🕐   AM / PM

transportation 🚶 🚴 🚗

washed hands before   yes - no

hand sanitizer before   yes - no

mask on you   yes - no

body temperature

air circulation   outdoors or inside

number of people

washed hands after   yes - no

hand sanitizer after   yes - no

PLACE and address   DATE:

your health:

NAMES include people you traveled with   **mask yes / no**

___

___

___

___

describe the social distancing

ARRIVAL TIME   AM / PM

DEPARTURE TIME   AM / PM

transportation

washed hands before   yes - no

hand sanitizer before   yes - no

mask on you   yes - no

body temperature

air circulation   outdoors or inside

number of people

washed hands after   yes - no

hand sanitizer after   yes - no

PLACE and address   DATE:

your health:

NAMES include people you traveled with   **mask yes / no**

___

___

___

___

describe the social distancing

ARRIVAL TIME   AM / PM

DEPARTURE TIME   AM / PM

transportation

washed hands before   yes - no

hand sanitizer before   yes - no

mask on you   yes - no

body temperature

air circulation   outdoors or inside

number of people

washed hands after   yes - no

hand sanitizer after   yes - no

PLACE and address

DATE:

your health:

NAMES include people you traveled with

mask yes / no

___

___

___

___

describe the social distancing

ARRIVAL TIME AM / PM

DEPARTURE TIME AM / PM

transportation

washed hands before   yes - no

hand sanitizer before   yes - no

mask on you   yes - no

body temperature

air circulation   outdoors or inside

number of people

washed hands after   yes - no

hand sanitizer after   yes - no

PLACE and address   **DATE:**

your health:

NAMES include people you traveled with   **mask yes / no**

___

___

___

___

describe the social distancing

ARRIVAL TIME 🕐	AM / PM
DEPARTURE TIME 🕐	AM / PM
transportation 🚶 🚴 🚗	
washed hands before	yes - no
hand sanitizer before	yes - no
mask on you	yes - no
body temperature	
air circulation	outdoors or inside
number of people	
washed hands after	yes - no
hand sanitizer after	yes - no

PLACE and address

DATE:

your health:

NAMES include people you traveled with

mask yes / no

___

___

___

___

describe the social distancing

ARRIVAL TIME AM / PM

DEPARTURE TIME AM / PM

transportation

washed hands before — yes - no

hand sanitizer before — yes - no

mask on you — yes - no

body temperature

air circulation — outdoors or inside

number of people

washed hands after — yes - no

hand sanitizer after — yes - no

PLACE and address   DATE:

your health:

NAMES include people you traveled with   **mask yes / no**

___

___

___

___

describe the social distancing

ARRIVAL TIME   AM / PM

DEPARTURE TIME   AM / PM

transportation

washed hands before   yes - no

hand sanitizer before   yes - no

mask on you   yes - no

body temperature

air circulation   outdoors or inside

number of people

washed hands after   yes - no

hand sanitizer after   yes - no

PLACE and address   DATE:

your health:

NAMES include people you traveled with

mask yes / no

___

___

___

___

describe the social distancing

ARRIVAL TIME 🕐	AM / PM
DEPARTURE TIME 🕐	AM / PM
transportation	
washed hands before	yes - no
hand sanitizer before	yes - no
mask on you	yes - no
body temperature	
air circulation	outdoors or inside
number of people	
washed hands after	yes - no
hand sanitizer after	yes - no

PLACE and address   DATE:

your health:

NAMES include people you traveled with   **mask yes / no**

___

___

___

___

describe the social distancing

ARRIVAL TIME 🕐   AM / PM

DEPARTURE TIME 🕐   AM / PM

transportation 🚶 🚴 🚗

washed hands before   yes - no

hand sanitizer before   yes - no

mask on you   yes - no

body temperature

air circulation   outdoors or inside

number of people

washed hands after   yes - no

hand sanitizer after   yes - no

PLACE and address

DATE:

your health:

NAMES include people you traveled with

mask yes / no

___

___

___

___

describe the social distancing

ARRIVAL TIME 🕐   AM / PM

DEPARTURE TIME 🕐   AM / PM

transportation

washed hands before   yes - no

hand sanitizer before   yes - no

mask on you   yes - no

body temperature

air circulation   outdoors or inside

number of people

washed hands after   yes - no

hand sanitizer after   yes - no

PLACE and address   DATE:

your health:

NAMES include people you traveled with   **mask yes / no**

___

___

___

___

describe the social distancing

ARRIVAL TIME 🕐   AM / PM

DEPARTURE TIME 🕐   AM / PM

transportation 🚶 🚴 🚗

washed hands before   yes - no

hand sanitizer before   yes - no

mask on you   yes - no

body temperature

air circulation   outdoors or inside

number of people

washed hands after   yes - no

hand sanitizer after   yes - no

PLACE and address   DATE:

your health:

NAMES include people you traveled with   **mask yes / no**

___

___

___

___

describe the social distancing

ARRIVAL TIME   AM / PM

DEPARTURE TIME   AM / PM

transportation

washed hands before   yes - no

hand sanitizer before   yes - no

mask on you   yes - no

body temperature

air circulation   outdoors or inside

number of people

washed hands after   yes - no

hand sanitizer after   yes - no

Made in the USA
Columbia, SC
27 June 2020